HEALTHY LIFESTYLES AND YOU

CLARICE INGRAHAM

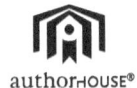

authorHOUSE®

AuthorHouse™
1663 Liberty Drive
Bloomington, IN 47403
www.authorhouse.com
Phone: 1-800-839-8640

First published by AuthorHouse 4/5/2011

ISBN: 978-1-4567-2672-0 (sc)
ISBN: 978-1-4567-2673-7 (e)
ISBN: 978-1-4567-2674-4 (dj)

Library of Congress Control Number: 2011900609

Printed in the United States of America

Any people depicted in stock imagery provided by Thinkstock are models, and such images are being used for illustrative purposes only. Certain stock imagery © Thinkstock.

This book is printed on acid-free paper.

ACKNOWLEDGEMENT

First and for most I thank the Good Lord for keeping me in a right frame of mind and seeing me through this course. I also want to express my heartfelt thanks to

- Pastor Strachan, W., for inspiring me to write this book.
- Rolle, Lessiah, my brother, for encouraging me to publish it.

May God graciously bless and keep all of you. A very special thank you is extended to the following persons, who provided invaluable assistance to the author.

- Mrs. Perpall, Erika and Forbes, Patrick for being there for me whenever I needed them.
- Last but not at all least, my immediate family members, for enduring all the hardship I have put them through.

TABLE OF CONTENTS

HEALTHY LIFESTYLE AND YOU

Being Healthy Is More Valuable Than Gold/Wealth

What is more precious than gold/wealth? Good health is not merely the absence of disease physically. It involves the body, mind and the spiritual wellbeing. It is the whole person. The good Lord had make mankind with the ability to make choices. We can choose healthy or unhealthy lifestyles. The human body consists of about 70% water. It is estimated that the daily water loss from the body by evaporation is about 2,000mls (perspiration /sweat). Water loss through urination average about 1,500 ml, other means, such as vomiting or diarrhoea averages 3,500 ml. Therefore we should drink 8 - 10 glasses (10ozs) glasses of potable water daily to maintain the water balance in the body. The Japanese Sickness Association has published the WATER TREATMENT which has attained 100% results in the cure of diseases such as:

1. Headache, Blood Pressure, Anemia, Paralysis, Epilepsy and Obesity.
2. Cough, Bronchitis, Asthma, Tuberculosis (TB).
3. Meningitis and any other disease connected with the liver and uterine.
4. Hyperacidity, Gastritis, Dysentery, Constipation, Diabetes and Files.
5. Any diseases connected with the eyes.
6. Irregular menstrual period of women, cancer of the uterus
7. Any disease connected with E.N.T. (ears, nose and throat).

METHOD OF TREATMENT

GET UP EARLY IN THE MORNING AND DRINK 4 GLASSES OF WATER (160 ML – 10 oz EACH /ROOM TEMPERATURE) BEFORE BRUSHING AND CLEANING TEETH

THEREAFTER

A. No solid or liquid to be taken up to 45 minutes except brushing teeth..
B. Normal food may be taken after 45 minutes.
C. Two (2) hours after breakfast, lunch or dinner you may eat anything.
D. After regular dinner, do not take any food before retiring.
E. Sick or old people, who find it difficult initially to drink 4 glasses of water at a time, may start with small quantities to be gradually increased to the recommended level of 4 glasses.

The above will definitely cure the disease of the sick person and will also ensure a healthy life for others. The treatment has proved that the following diseases may be cured within the period stated against them. They are as follows:

1. Hypertension   30 days
2. Gastric problem   10 days
3. Diabetes   30 days
4. Constipation   10 days
5. Cancer   6 months
6. TB   3 months

Those who are suffering from Arthritis should do this experiment for one week, three times a day, thereafter once a day. There is no side effect. For the first few days, you might have to pass water more regularly.

CREATE BALANCE......

There are many health benefits of eating a diet rich with fruits and vegetables. Besides being colourful and attractive they are loaded with fibre, potassium, foliate, vitamins A and C (antioxidants) and phytochemicals. They are also low in calories, fat, and sodium. Combining a variety of colons with whole grains, nuts, low fat dairy products and physical activities and exercise promote health and may substantially reduce the risk of hypertension, diabetes, cancer and heart disease. We need 5 to 9 servings of fruits and vegetables every day.

Eat/Drink Your Colours Everyday!

When you're shopping, planning your meals or eating out - "Think Colour."

Go for red for a healthy heart!

Powerful ingredients: Lycopene, Anthocyanins

1. For good heart health
2. For a healthy urinary tract
3. Improve your memory
4. Lower your risk(s) of some cancers
5. Improve your brain power.

Red apples	Raspberries	Tomatoes
Cherries	Strawberries, Rhubarb	Cranberries
Watermelon	Red onions	Red grapes
Beets Radishes	Red peppers	Pears
Pomegranates	Pink/red grapefruit	

Go for Green for vitality!

Powerful Ingredients: Lutein, insoles.

1. Get radiant skin
2. Improve your memory
3. Increase your longevity
4. For a healthy urinary tract
5. Strengthen your immune system
6. Lower your risk(s) of some cancers

Green beans	Okra	Broccoli
Green peas	Limes	Green apples
Avocados	Asparagus	Endives
Kiwi fruit	Cabbage	String beans
Lettuce	Green grapes	Green peppers
Zucchini	Spinach	
Brussels sprouts	Honeydew melon	

Get White & Brown for Wellness!

Powerful ingredients: allicin (onions & garlic)

- Normalize your cholesterol levels
- Promote heart health
- Strengthen your immune system
- Lower your risk(s) for some cancers

Onions	Sour sop	White sweet potatoes
Garlic	Sapodilla	Mushrooms
Tamarind	Mamee	Cauliflower
Eddoes	Cassava	Ginger
Bananas	Cocoa plums	Sugar apple
Jelly coconut		

Stay Young with Purple & Blue!

Powerful Ingredients: Anthocyanins. Phenolics

1. Sharpen your eye sight
2. Strengthen your bones and teeth
3. Improve your memory
4. Strengthen your immune system
5. Lower your risk(s) for some cancers

Blueberries	Egg plants	Plums
Red Cabbage	Figs	Red grapes
Raisins	Purple potatoes	Prunes
Cocoa plums	Pigeon plums	Black currants

Power Up With Yellow & Orange

Powerful Ingredients: Carotenoids, Bioflavonoid, Antioxidant, Vitamin C

1. Get radiant glowing skin
2. Strengthen your heart

3. Sharpen your eye sight
4. Strengthen your immune system
5. Lower your risk(s) of some cancers

Pineapple	Papaya	Peaches
Cantaloupe	Hog plums	Apricots
Nectarines	Squash	Carrots
Scarlet plums	Star fruit	Tangerine
Oranges	Pumpkins	Mangos
Sweet potatoes	Corn	

Handy Portion Guide

Your hands, they're always with you, and they're always the same size Your hands can be very useful in estimating appropriate portions. When planning a meal, use these portions

CARBOHYDRATES – (grains and starches): Choose an amount the size of your 2 fists. For fruit, use 1 fist.

PROTEIN: Choose an amount the size of the palm of your hand and the thickness of your little finger.

VEGETABLES: Choose as much as you can hold in both hands. Choose low-carbohydrate vegetables (e.g. green or yellow beans, broccoli, and lettuce).

FAT: Limit fat to an amount the size of the tip of your thumb.

Remember your plate should be dived into 3 imaginary portions – ½ (half) for your vegetables, ¼ (quarter) for your starch (potato, rice or pasta). For your protein the other ¼ (quarter) of your plate should consist of (fish, lean meat, chicken, beans, lentils.) Remember you should always have a glass of water and a fruit with meal

Health Tips to remember
The Portion Plate
½ of your plate should be fruits and vegetables (one cup of fruits or vegetables = the size of a baseball.

¼ starch/whole grains
A medium potato = the size of a computer mouse
The width of a pancake = the size of a cd.
A slice of bread = the size of an audio cassette

¼ protein/lean meat
One serving of meat = the size of a deck of cards

Fat, oils & sweets – Use sparingly.

Vitamins & Supplements to live by – Guide for your Health ...

Alpha Lipoic Acid – Antioxidant with metabolic function/ The universal Antioxidant, services a variety of important functions in the body, including helping to metabolize sugar, especially in muscles where it promotes energy.
1. A powerful antioxidant that helps neutralizes free radicals.
2. Helps metabolize sugar.
3. Beneficial for liver health.
4. Helps skin look healthier and more radiant.

Vitamin E – The most effective Fat-Soluble Antioxidant E is for everybody. Found in many food sources including nuts, seeds, egg yolks and peanut butter.
1. Helps fight against free radicals and oxidative stress.
2. Promotes circulatory and metabolic function.
3. Helps maintain a healthy immune system.
4. Nutritionally supports cardiovascular health and healthy blood vessels.
5. Supports prostate health.

Selenium – A Trace Mineral with widespread benefits, necessary for good health – food sources such as crab, liver, poultry and wheat.

Selenium provides powerful antioxidant support, promotes immune system health and an integral part of the protein structure in teeth.

1. Provides powerful antioxidant support.
2. Promotes immune system health.
3. Is an integral part of protein structure in the teeth.
4. Assists in regulating the body's metabolic rate.
5. Assists with proper utilization of iodine in thyroid function.
6. Support prostrate health.

Calcium- Major Mineral, well-being for bones and teeth.

1. Responsible for strong bones and bone well-being
2. Provides the building blocks for strong teeth.
3. Helps to maintain the health of the, muscles and nerves.
4. A major mineral essential for nutrition.\

Vitamin D – The Sunshine Vitamin, a sunny supplement. A lack of exposure to sunlight may reduce Vitamin D levels in the body, especially in the winter.

1. Involved in proper bone mineralization.
2. Works with calcium to maintain healthy bones and teeth in adults.
3. Assists in maintaining a healthy immune system.
4. Helps to increase calcium absorption.

Bone care; Magnesium – For Nerves, Bones, Cells and more, a major mineral for strong bones.

1. Crucial for cell formation
2. Promotes healthy bones.
3. Involved in protein formation and nerve impulses.
4. May work with vitamin B-6 to help promote menstrual health.
5. Helpful for occasional muscle tension related to exercise.

Digestive Health- Acidophilus – Enrich your body with beneficial bacteria, naturally found in the intestinal tract. Known as a 'probiotic', these bacteria can also be found in yogurt. These bacteria support the digestive system by having a favourable environment for the absorption of nutrients.

1. Nutritionally supports digestive system.
2. Supports normal immune function.
3. Supports healthy intestinal flora.
4. A normal constituent of the vaginal flora, where it contributes to the maintenance of a healthy acidic environment.

Echinacea
Immune System Herb
1. #1 herb for helping to maintain healthy immune function
2. Promotes the body's natural defence system
3. Contains beneficial polysaccharides and phytosterols
4. Popular during times of seasonal change

Ester-C
The Better Vitamin C
1. Helps support immune system health, good vision, cardiovascular health, and healthy joints.
2. Functions as an antioxidant that fights cell-damaging free radicals in the body.
3. Promotes enhanced absorption and delayed excretion of vitamin C.

Zinc
Body of Work
1. Contributes to skin health
2. Important for testosterone synthesis
3. Assists in the formation of DNA
4. Plays a vital role in RNA transcription, cell division and growth, and protein formation

Chondroitin Sulphates
Joint and Connective Tissue Nutrition
1. Provides structural support for cartilage and joints
2. Lubricates and cushions joints
3. Supports mobility, flexibility, and comfortable joint movement
4. Helps re-new and revitalize cartilage

Glucosamine Sulphates
Supplement Your Joint Strength
1.   A key structural component in cartilage
2.   Nourishes and revitalizes the cellular components within joints
3.   Is one of the top three structural components found in popular joint support products
4.   Acts as a lubricant in order to nutritionally support healthy joints for comfortable movement

MSM (Methylsulfonylmethane)
One of Joint Health's Top Three
1.   Vital in the formation of collagen, connective tissue, and healthy joint cartilage
2.   Supports the cellular components within your joints
3.   Supports joint comfort
4.   As an organic source of sulfur, MSM supplies a vital ingredient that nourishes joints

Ginkgo Biloba
Mental Focus and the World's Oldest Living Tree
1.   Helps maintain healthy circulation to the arms, legs and brain
2.   Helps improve memory
3.   Contains antioxidant properties that help fight free radicals in the body
4.   Supports brain function and mental focus

Lecithin
Don't Forget Your Lecithin
1.   Promotes mental function and nerve cell health
2.   Supports cell growth and function
3.   Contributes to the health of the nervous system
4.   An important natural source of choline, inositol and linoleic acid

Neuro-PS.
(Phosphatidylserine)
1.   Supports brain function
2.   Has a positive influence on memory and sharpens mental focus

3. Promotes the thought process
4. Perfect for occasional mild memory problems associated with aging

Lycopene
Heart, Immune System and Prostate Support
1. Supports prostate and immune system health
2. Provides antioxidant support Promotes heart health

Saw Palmetto
The prostate and Urinary Health Herb
1. Promotes both prostate and urinary health in men
2. Contains beneficial phytochemicals and polysaccharides

CLA (Conjugated Linoleic Acid)
Diet Support from a Flower
1. A form of the essential fatty acid Linoleic Acid
2. Provides exercise and dieting support
3. Helps promote a healthy body composition

Cinnamon
Aromatic, Tasty and Good for You
1. Supports sugar metabolism
2. Contains valuable terpenoids, including eugenol and cinnamaldehyde

Green Tea
Feel Good Going Green
1. Provides antioxidant support
2. Helps boost metabolism
3. Promotes heart and skin health
4. Supports thermogenesis

L-Carnitine
Fuel for the Heart
1. Assists in energy metabolism
2. Helps make energy available to the heart

3. Plays an essential role in making fatty acids available for muscle tissue

Melatonin
Natural Way to Quality Sleep
1. Supports a relaxed mood
2. Helps to promote restful sleep patterns and calm, tranquil rest
3. Nutritionally supports sound sleep

St. John's Wort
Relaxation Give your mood a boost
1. Promotes mental well-being and a peaceful mood.
2. Relieves occasional anxiety and every day stress.
3. Supports a feeling of tranquillity, allowing for calm and relax mental state.
4. Boosts an extensive range of flavonoids.

Valerian
Sleep Cycle Harmony
5. Supports calm tranquil rest
6. Works in harmony with your natural cycle to promote relaxation.
7. Supports a relaxed state of mind.

Creatine Powder
Natural Choice for Muscle Support
1. Supports muscle mass and strength
2. Plays a key role in energy transfer within skeletal muscles
3. Can help increase strength, power, and support muscle size
4. Helps muscles during the recovery phase after high-intensity exercise

DHEA (Dehydroepiandrorterone)
Metabolize the sugar
1. Promotes sugar metabolism.
2. May promote well-being, mood and relaxation.

Glutamine
Muscle fuel
1. Support protein metabolism while providing fuel for muscles.
2. May promote replenishment of muscle glycogen stores after exercise.
3. Plays a role in the proper functioning of the gastrointestinal tract.
4. Important for the immune system.

Protein Supplements
A resource for body function
1. Protein supplementation can help to increase strength and support recovery from exercise.
2. Assists in normal growth and development.
3. Plays a role in constructing and maintaining the critical structures and functions of the body.

Black Cohosh
Natural Menopausal Relief
1. Supports female health around the time of menopause
2. Helps alleviate hot flashes and night sweats
3. Helps support the physical and emotional changes that occur in a woman's body over time

Cranberry
Urinary tract health/Helps the flow when you go
1. Supports urinary tract health in men and women.
2. Removes unwanted compounds from the urinary tract.
3. Promotes the healthy flow of urine.

Evening Primrose Oil
For women of all ages/Natural; Support for women's health.
1. Provides nutritional support for women with PMS.
2. Promotes menstrual health.
3. A Natural source of Gamma Linoleic Acid (GLA).

Soy Isoflavones
"Soy" Good for you
1. Help to maintain cholesterol levels that are already in the normal range.
2. Help relieve the physical changes related to menopause.
3. Contribute to bone health by helping to support calcium metabolism.
4. Beneficial in supporting prostate health in men.

Heart Health
Your heart loves **Co Q-10**
1. It is essential for energy promotion at the cellular level.
2. It helps the body convert food to energy.
3. It is an antioxidant that fights cell-damaging free radicals in the body.
4. It is a powerful weapon in supporting heart health.
5. Taking statin drugs for high cholesterol can deplete Co Q-10 levels in the body.

Fish Oils
Omega-3s from the Seas
1. Fish oils play a major role in cardiovascular health.
2. It supports the immune and nervous systems.
3. It is vital for normal cell growth.
4. It may help support healthy joints.

Flaxseed Oil
Flaxseed oil is one of the most concentrated plant sources of Omega-3s.
1. It contains Alpha Linolenic Acid and Linoleic Acid.
2. Flaxseed naturally contains heart healthy nutrients.
3. It can support healthy cholesterol levels that are already within the normal range.

Garlic
Garlic does your heart good.
1. It promotes heart and cardiovascular health.

2. It helps to maintain cholesterol levels that are already within the normal range.
3. It has antioxidant properties.

The Master Cleanser or the lemonade Diet

The purpose
To dissolve and eliminate toxins and congestion that has formed in any part of the body.

To - cleanse the kidneys and the digestive system.

To- purify the glands and cells throughout the entire body.

To - eliminate all unusable waste and hardened material in the joints and muscles.

To - relieve pressure and irritation in the nerves, arteries and blood vessels.

To - build a healthy blood stream.

To - keep youth and elasticity regardless of our years.

When to use
When sickness developed - for all acute and chronic conditions.

When the - digestive system needs a rest and a cleaning.

When overweight has become a problem.

When - better assimilation and building of body tissues is needed.

How often should you use the diet?
Follow the diet for a minimum of 10 days or more - up to 40 days and may be safely followed for extremely serious cases. The diet has all the nutrition needed during this time. Three to four times a year will do wonders for keeping the body in a normal healthy condition. The diet may be undertaken more frequently for serious conditions.

How to make
2: Table spoons of lemon juice (approx; half a lemon).

2: Table spoons of genuine maple syrup (grade A, B, or C, not maple flavoured sugar syrup).

1/10: Table spoon of Cayenne pepper. (Add pepper to taste).

- Water, medium hot/room temperature (spring or purified).

Combine the lime juice, maple syrup and cayenne pepper in a 10 ounce glass and fill with purified water. Use fresh lemons or limes only, never canned or frozen.

The maple syrup is a balanced form of positive and negative form of sugar and must be used.

Maple syrup has a variety of minerals and vitamins. The minerals and vitamin content varies according to the area where the trees grow and the mineral content of the soil. The maple syrup from Vermont contains sodium; potassium; calcium; magnesium; iron; copper; phosphorus; sulphur; chlorine; and silicon. Vitamin A, B1, B2, B6, C, Nicotinic acid and Pantothenic acid are also present in the syrup.

Special Instructions for Diabetic
The lemonade with Molasses is an ideal way to correct diabetic deficiency.

Consult your doctor before undertaking the diet.

For best results, follow the direction carefully. The molasses supplies the necessary elements for the pancreas to produce insulin. As the necessary elements are supplied to the pancreas, the amount of insulin taken may be gradually reduced - as an example.

The First Day - use a scant table spoon of molasses to each glass of lemonade and reduce insulin by 10 units. Daily from then on reduce the insulin as you increase the molasses to 2 full table spoons per glass. When this proportion has been reached the insulin can normally be eliminated; then replace the molasses with 2 table spoons of maple syrup in each glass. Make certain to make regular checks of sugar level in the urine and blood to satisfy yourself and eliminate any possible fear. Vita Flex and colour therapy may be used to advantage to stimulate the liver, pancreas, and spleen and thus insure proper use of the minerals supplied. Many people have found they no longer have the need for insulin. They must be sure to follow every detail of recommended diet as explained.

How much to drink

Take about 6 to 12 glasses of lemonade daily during the day. As you get hungry, have another glass of lemonade. NO OTHER FOOD SHOULD BE TAKEN DURING THE PERIOD OF THE DIET. As this is a complete balance minerals and vitamins, one does not suffer the pangs of hunger. Do not use vitamin pills. All solid food is turned into a liquid state before it can be carried by the blood to the cells of the body. The lemonade is already a food in liquid form.

For those who are overweight, less maple syrup may be taken. For those who are underweight and worried about losing more weight, REMEMBER, the only thing you can possibly loose, are mucus, waste and disease. Healthy tissues will not be eliminated; many people who need to gain weight usually do so near the end of the diet period. Never vary the amount of lemon juice per glass. About 6 glasses of lemonade per day is enough for those wishing to reduce, extra water may be taken as desired.

Lecithin

Known as the furnace of the body

Lecithin was discovered in 1881, and extensively researched by William McDonald in the 1930s. Doctors were giving their patients four to six tablespoons of glandular lecithin a day for up to 10 years. It was called "the furnace of the body" because they believed it burned the fat and cholesterol which supplies heat and energy for the body. It was discovered that persons who have had heart attacks due to booked veins, were advised to take three tablespoons of lecithin granules daily for several weeks. These persons were scheduled for cardiac bypass surgery, but after taking the lecithin the surgery was not necessary. On examination the veins were perfectly clear.

It was discovered that Lecithin;
1. Lowers and control blood pressure
2. Improves memory
3. Protect cells from damage by oxidation
4. Help the liver to absorb thiamine and the intestine absorb vitamin A.

It is important that the elderly take lecithin because it prevents arteriosclerosis and cardiovascular diseases, increases brain function, and promotes energy.

5. It helps to repair the liver when it is damaged by alcohol.
6. It relieves hot flashes during the menopausal changes
7. 7 It alleviates mood swings and palpation.
8. Helps to lose weight and prevents constipation.
9. Normalized cholesterol

Organic Unrefined Virgin Coconut Oil
Falls under the "Miraculous" category

The health-giving properties contained in coconut oil are overwhelming Take one tablespoon in the morning and a tablespoon in late afternoon. Do this every day for thirty days, here is what you find.

1. High blood pressure will be a thing of the past.
2. Circulation problems vanish.
3. Mood swings are gone. Depression lifted.
4. Constipation cured
5. Arthritis pain reduced or totally eliminative.
6. Cancer in remission
7. Cholesterol normalized
8. Acid reflux and heart burn diminished or gone forever.
9. If you are overweight you will probably lose up to ten pounds.

Add Activity to your life
Regular exercise and physical activity can:

1. Help build strong bones and muscles
2. Increase energy.
3. Help you lose and maintain a healthy weight
4. Help prevent certain diseases/conditions in the future, such as heart disease, arthritis and type 2 diabetes
5. Increase your strength and endurance.
6. Help you sleep better
7. Help you feel and look good.
8. Help improve your self esteem and be more self-confident
9. Help you learn better and are alert.
10. Help you to be more flexible.

Tips for Healthy lifestyle Activities

- Use the stairs instead of the elevator or escalator
- Walk briskly.
- Park your car far from entrances.
- Find something to do instead of sitting around the house.
- Watch less television or do exercises while watching television.
- Go for a walk after a meal instead of sitting or lying down.
- Choose a hobby that requires body movement.
- Exercise for at least 1/2 hour 4 times per week to maintain a healthy weight & at least 45 minutes 5 times per week to lose weight.

You and your health

Clarice Ingraham, RN, RM, CHN, appreciates the assistance of the following -

http://www.modelherbs.com/uploads/news-image001.jpg, (front cover page, fruits picture on the) Nutrition Unit, Department of Public Health/Ministry of Health and Social Development, April 2006.

Textbook of Medical/Surgical Nursing - seventh edition by Brunner, Emerson, Ferguson and Suddarth.

Puritan's Pride leaflet information 2008.

"The Master Cleanser", or Lemonade Diet" - By Stanley Burroughs 1941.

"Medical miracle with water" - By the (JSA) Japanese sickness Association.

More Natural Cures Revealed. By Kevin Trudeau

Appendices - www.paledodetonline.com/image bp3.blogger.com/.../ s400/fruit-marked.jpg and vegetables and fruits pictures from Improve your mental health by Joy Baver Dietician.

Appendices

Portion size/amount

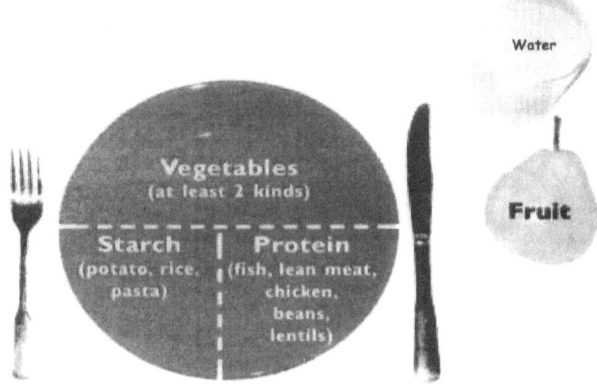

The portion plate

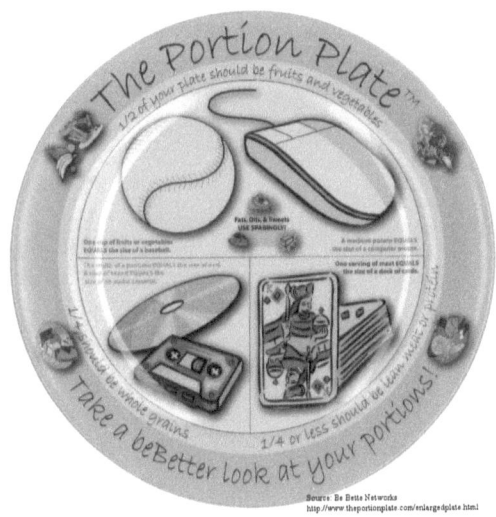

Vegetables

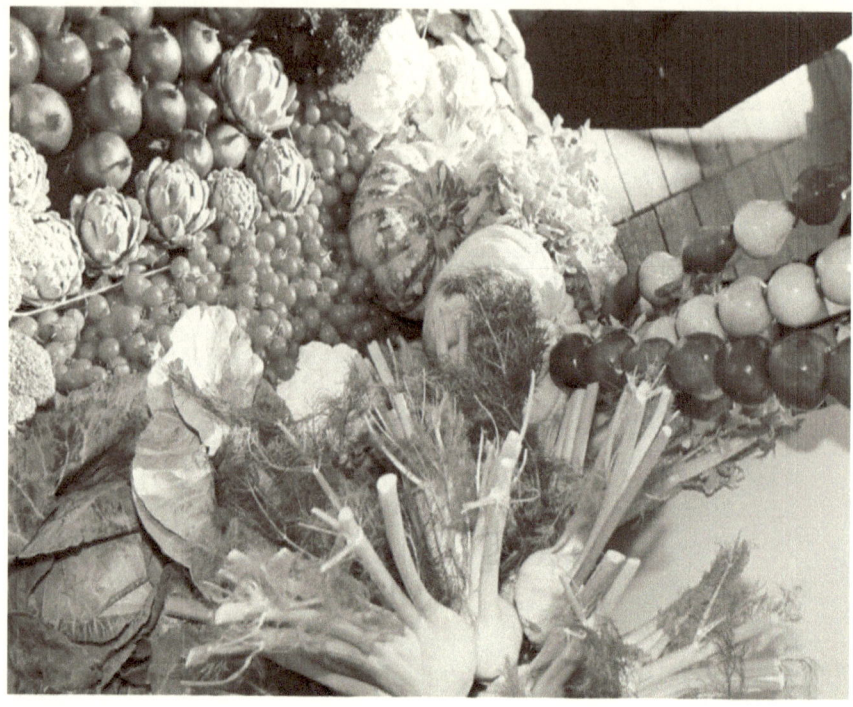

Red onions, Asparagus, Tomatoes, Broccolis, Cabbages, Cauliflowers, Pumpkins, Mushrooms, Brussels sprouts, Celeries, Green and Red Apples

Dry Coconut

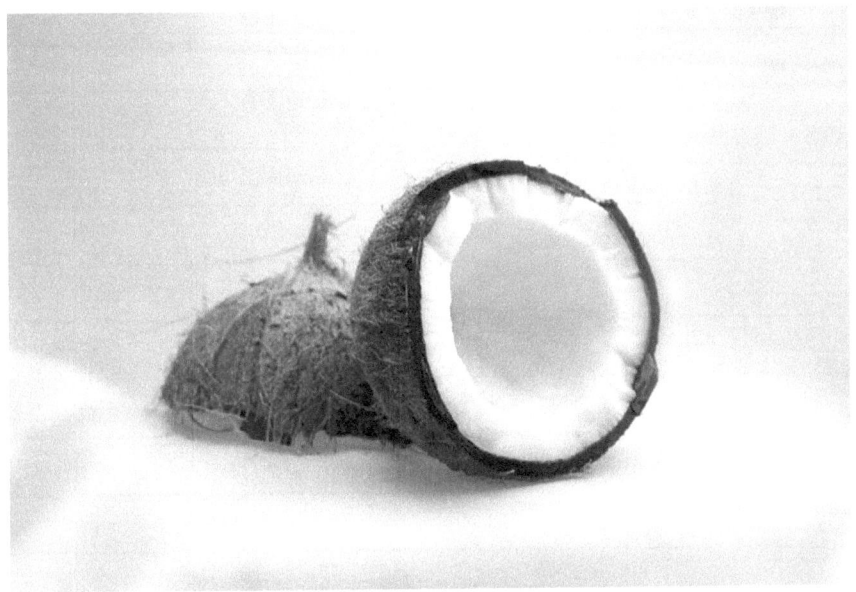

Notes

Notes

Notes

Notes

Notes

Notes

Notes

Notes

Notes

Notes

Notes

Notes

Notes

Notes

Notes

Notes

Notes

Notes

Notes

Notes

Notes

Notes

Notes

Notes

Notes

Notes

Notes

Notes

Notes

Notes

Notes

Notes

Notes

Notes

Notes

Notes

Notes

Notes

Notes

Notes

Notes

Notes

Notes

Notes

Notes

Notes

Notes

Notes

Notes

Notes

Notes

Notes

Notes

Notes

Notes

Notes

Notes

Notes

Notes

Notes

Notes

Notes

Notes

Notes

Notes

Notes

Notes

Notes

Notes

Notes

Notes

Notes

Notes

Notes

Notes

Notes

Notes

Notes

Notes

Notes